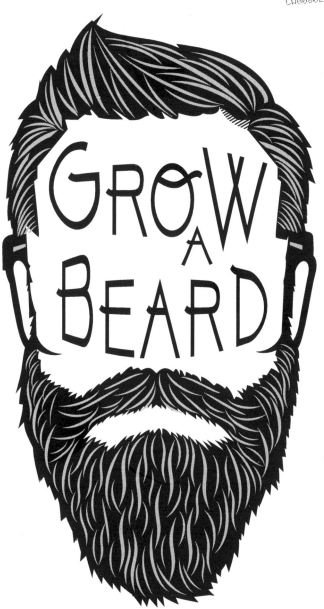

How to Grow a Beard

Copyright © Hamish McDuff 2022

First Edition February 2022

HOW

TO

GROW

A

BEARD

HAMISH MCDUFF

CONTENTS

INTRODUCTION

Are you frustrated with your fuzzy beard growth?

Want to get that manly look but don't know where to start?

This book is your complete guide to growing and grooming the beard you've always wanted. We'll start by looking at where beards began, then we'll go through how to manage the awkward growing phase.

Once you're feeling confident with your new bearded look, you can groom yourself into one of the many beard styles we've included in the book!

Now, it's grow time...

HOW TO GROW A BEARD

A SHORT HISTORY OF BEARDS

Beards have had different meanings throughout the ages. Let's look at some landmark moments for male facial hair.

CAVEMAN TIMES

Beards were grown to keep the face warm,

And for protection against fist fights!

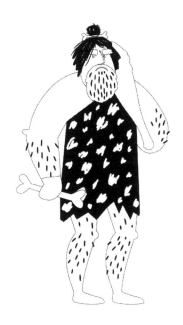

ANCIENT EYGPT

It was possible to buy yourself a fake beard made of gold!

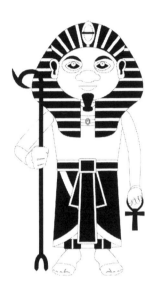

ANCIENT INDIA

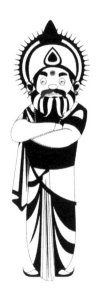

Long beards were a sign of wisdom.

They were a prized currency and could be snipped off to pay a debt if needed.

ANCIENT GREECE

Beards were a sign of honour. The Greeks took pride in their beards and even loved to curl them with tongs. If they misbehaved, their curls were snipped off as punishment!

Beards took a hit when Alexander the Great came along in 345 BCE. He decided having a beard that could be pulled on in battle was too much of a risk. He therefore declared that all beards be shaved for national safety!

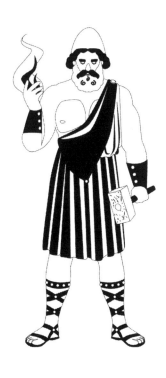

ROMANS

The Romans were ahead of the trend in short-beard fashion. They had realised that having a long beard was probably unhygienic, and encouraged razors to be used frequently.

If you were lucky, you'd have a slave to shave your beard for you. As shaving became more popular, barber shops were opened up so that everyone could get a slice of the action.

Meanwhile, philosophers didn't follow the trend and kept hold of their long beards (probably for stroking while thinking).

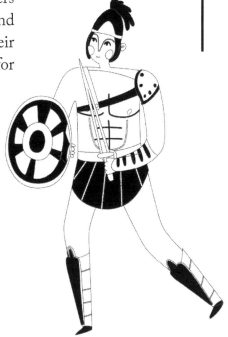

7TH CENTURY

In England, most men were bearded until the start of Christianity in the 7th century. The church wasn't a fan of a hairy face, so all Anglo Saxons were forced to shave off their pride and joy.

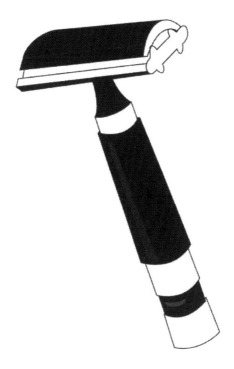

There was an exception for male royalty, though, who could show off a tasteful moustache. But in 1066, they had to keep up with Norman fashions and shave them clean off.

Beards didn't come back into fashion until the 1500s. By this time, men could try out whatever style they fancied.

1600

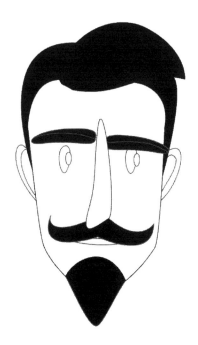

By 1600 people were taking their beards seriously.

The pointy Vandyke beard was popular, and men would use wax to form the shape.

There were even gadgets on the market to protect the shape of your moustache and beard while you slept!

VIKINGS

The Vikings took great pride in their beards and used them to spark fear wherever they went.

They grew them to great volume and length and even styled them with braids.

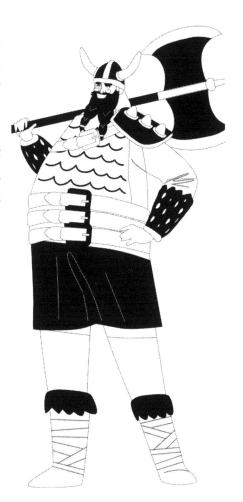

Beards and facial hair have always been important in battle. In the 18th century, French soldiers had specific looks depending on their roles - sometimes, growing a big moustache or a goatee was compulsory to fit in with the rest of the troop!

The British army also made moustaches compulsory between 1860 and 1916, but beards had to be clean shaven.

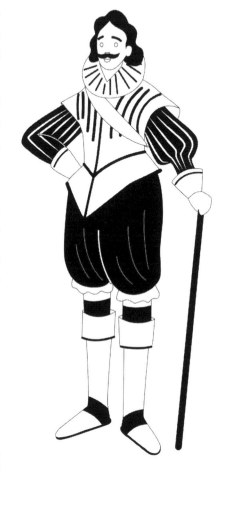

18TH CENTURY

◼ MODERN DAY

Today, beards are back and are more popular with the modern man than ever before.

Our ancestors have made facial hair look so effortless - but how does a gentleman get that irresistible masculine look today?

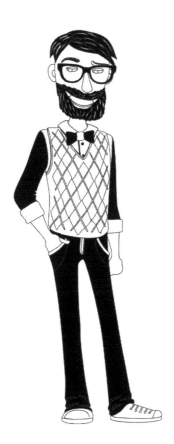

ARE YOU GETTING MORE
BUMFLUFF THAN BRISTLES?

LET'S BUST THESE MYTHS
ABOUT BEARD GROWTH SO
THAT YOU CAN GO FORTH AND
GROW THAT VIKING BEARD.

3 BEARD GROWING MYTHS

1. RUBBING YOUR BEARD CAN MAKE IT GROW FASTER

Unfortunately, constantly touching your beard with your hands is more likely to cause spots or ingrown hairs than help its growth. By all means, rub in a good moisturiser daily, but otherwise it's best to keep your oily hands away from your face.

2. LEAVE IT TO GROW FOR 6 WEEKS

Although it might be tempting to just leave your beard to its thing, without regular maintenance your growth will be weak and unhealthy. In the growing phase, it's important to use beard shampoo, oils and moisturiser so that your hair grows strong.

3. SHAVING WILL MAKE YOUR FACIAL HAIR GROW BIGGER AND THICKER

Despite what you may have heard, shaving everything off is not the secret to a thick and luscious bearded look. Take it slow and look after the hair you have - with proper grooming you'll be able to work towards your desired look without going bare faced to start with.

PART I

THE GROWING PHASE

THE SECRET WEAPON: TESTOSTERONE

Why can some men grow beards more easily than others? And why do women and children not have the same talent? The answer is testosterone, the sex hormone produced by men in the testicles.

While some men have slightly more testosterone than others, it is possible to boost your levels with proper exercise, diet and sleep. Males can also take hormone supplements where testosterone levels are especially low, but this should not be a usual course of action and should only be done after consulting with a medical professional.

GETTING PAST THE AWKWARD PHASE

During the first two or three weeks of growing a beard, you might doubt your decision. Not only will you have a new appearance to contend with, but you might also find yourself with an itchy, dry chin.

Don't give up!

You'll make it through by following these rules:
- Don't scratch
- Keep your skin moisturised
- Keep your new beard clean by using a special beard wash
- Use a beard oil to soothe the new hairs as they come through

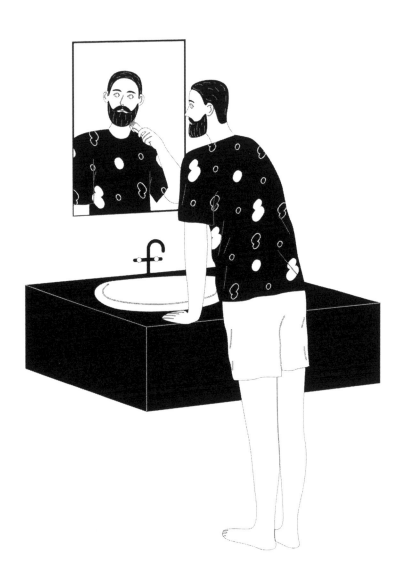

5 TOP TIPS FOR BEARD GROWTH

1. BE PATIENT

2. MOISTURISE

3. PRACTICE A HEALTHY LIFESTYLE

4. MAINTAIN A GROOMING ROUTINE

5. TRIM REGULARLY

PART 2

STYLING YOUR BEARD

Once your beard is growing freely, the style options are endless.Depending on the vibe you're going for, you can show off your new bearded look in the a range of styles - why not try out the butler, aristocrat or philosopher?

Achieving these styles will take time and patience, so don't be dissapointed if you don't get there straight away. Using the tools and knowledge in this book you'll be able to effectively groom, grow and maintain that sexy bearded look in no time.

Use our style inspiration guide to shape your facial hair into the look you've always dreamed of.

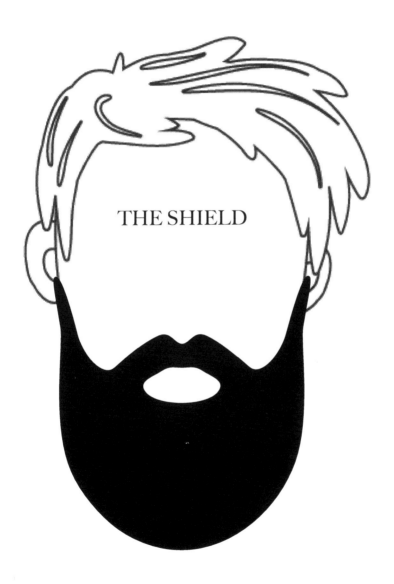

THE SHIELD

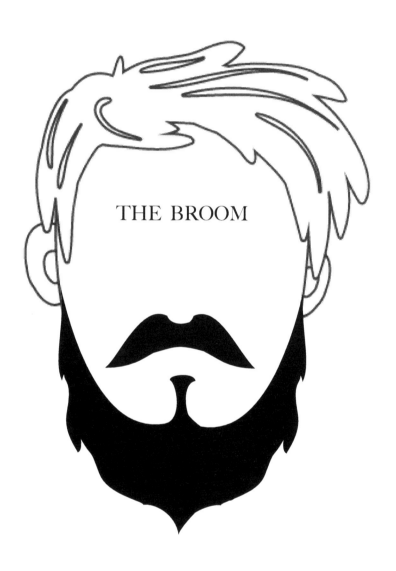

THE BROOM

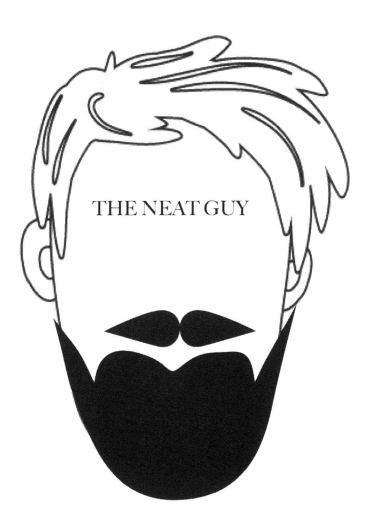

THE NEAT GUY

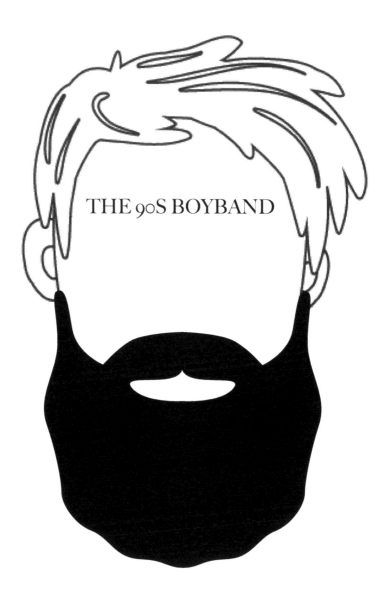

THE 90S BOYBAND

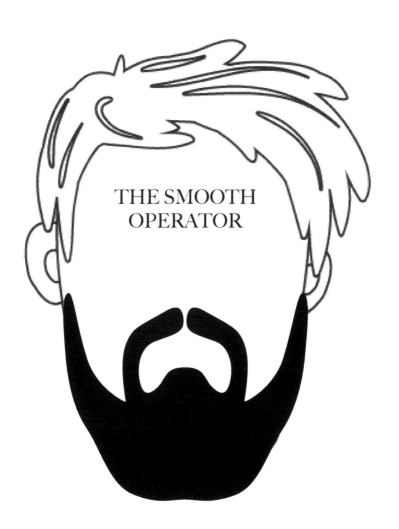

THE SMOOTH
OPERATOR

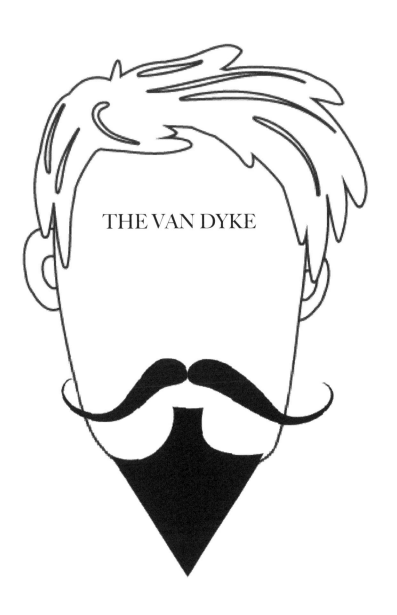

THE VAN DYKE

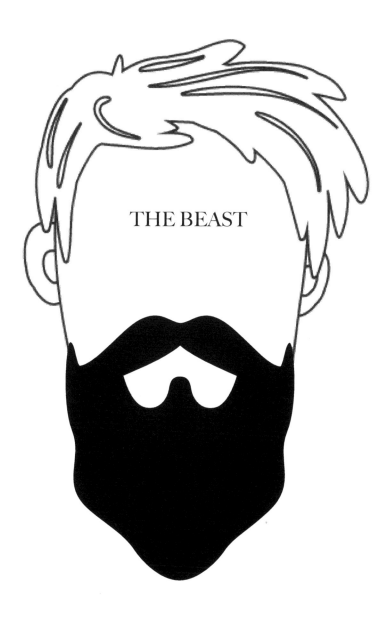

THE BEAST

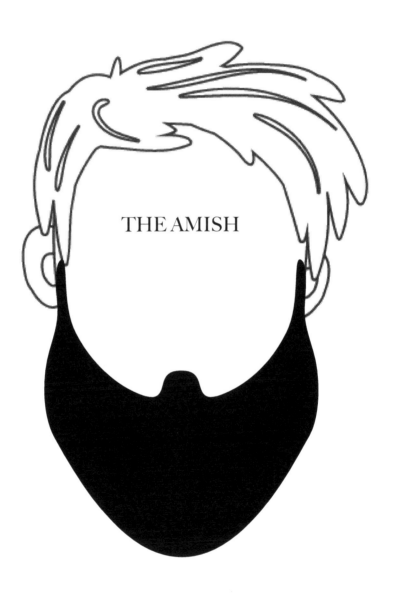

THE AMISH

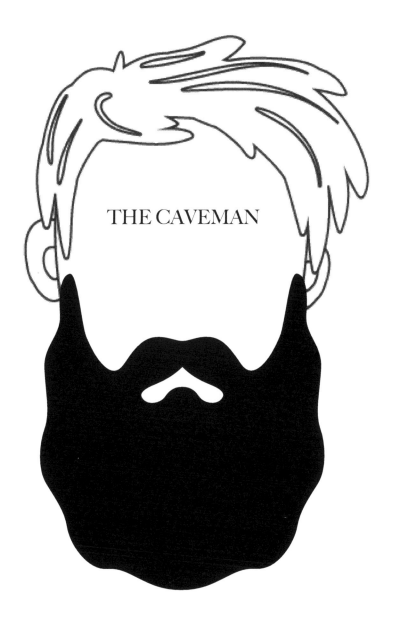

THE CAVEMAN

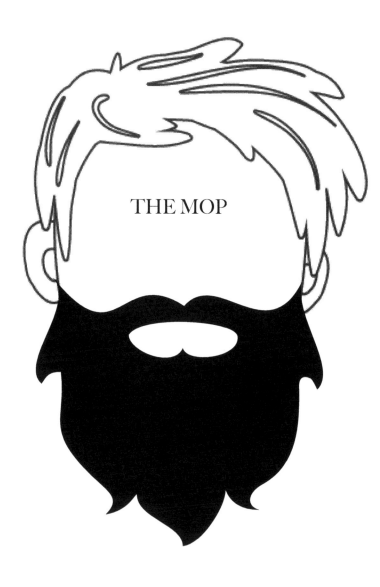

THE MOP

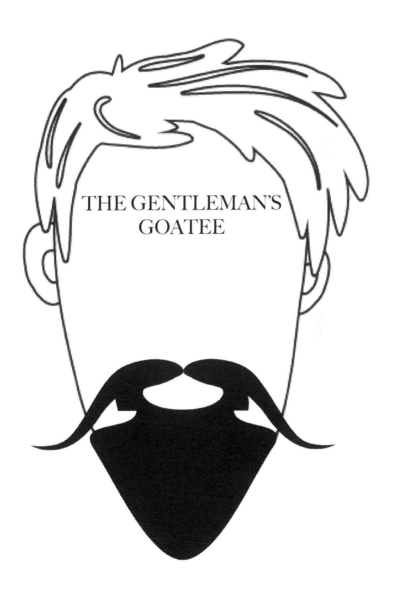

THE GENTLEMAN'S GOATEE

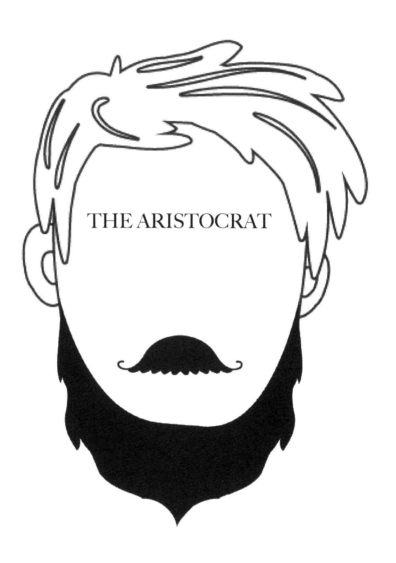

THE ARISTOCRAT

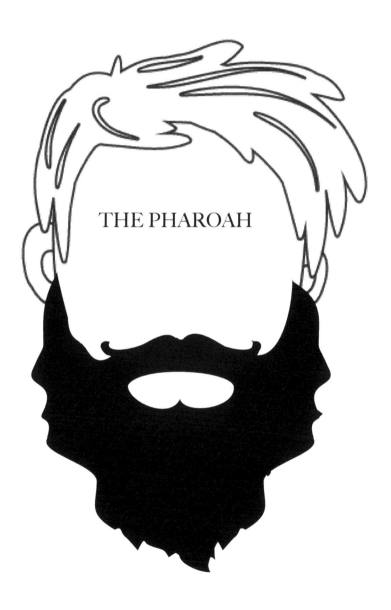

THE PHAROAH

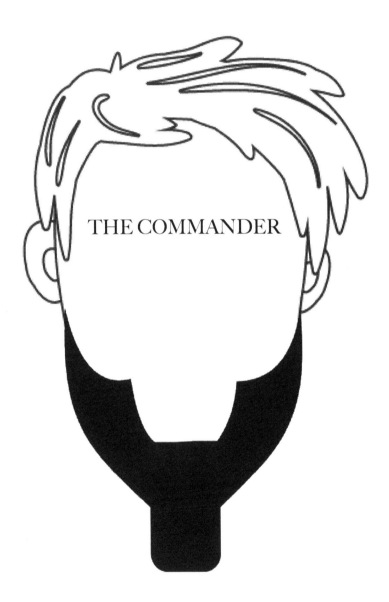

THE COMMANDER

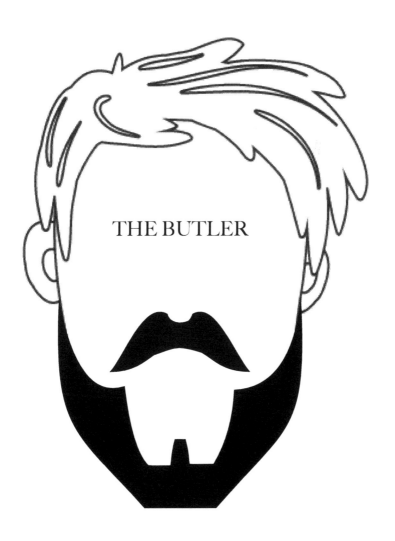

THE BUTLER

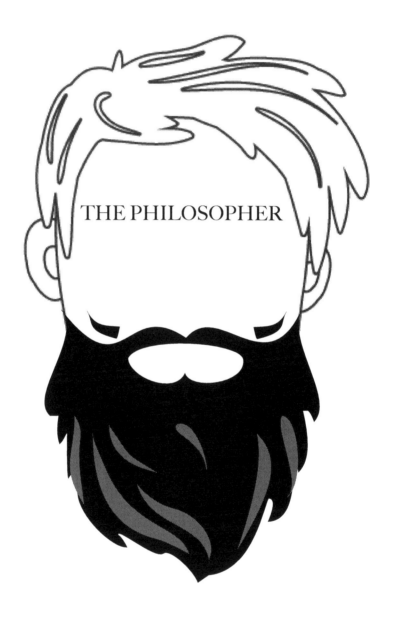

THE PHILOSOPHER

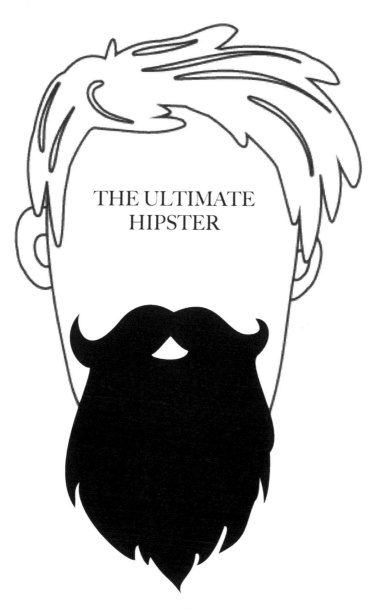

THE ULTIMATE
HIPSTER

PART 3

LIFE
WITH
A BEARD

HOW TO EAT

To avoid ending up looking like Roald Dahl's Mr Twit, you'll practice eating neatly. Keeping your beard well groomed will help you avoid any embarrassing bits getting stuck.

Here are our handy tips for eating with a beard:

- Open wide
- Use a knife and fork for messy things like pizza
- Avoid crumbly foods like croissants or flapjacks
- Carry a small beard comb to brush out any unwanted crumbs

HOW TO KISS

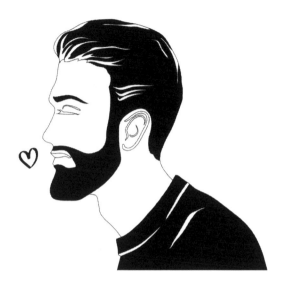

So you've grown a beard to look sexy, right? But how do you get intimate with your partner without leaving a nasty rash or giving them a mouth full of hair?

Keeping your beard properly combed and moisturised will ensure that you stay irresistible.

Taming your moustache is the most important thing before you pucker up. Trim the hair so that it doesn't fall over your mouth, or style it out of the way with some wax. You want to make sure that your lips are easily accessible!

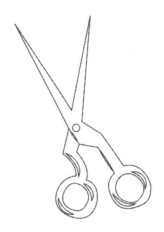

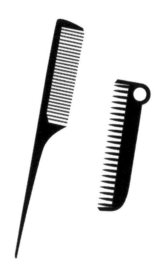

YOUR GROOMING ROUTINE

A QUICK GUIDE TO KEEPING YOUR BEARD IN SHAPE:

Brush your beard every morning. Getting into this habit will help you start the day looking neat.

Trim your beard. Once or twice a week, you'll want to grab a pair of sharp scissors and cut away any bits that look too long or too thick. Visit a barber or ask a friend to trim under your neck.

Wash your beard each time that you shower, preferably daily. Use a separate beard shampoo and conditioner to keep the hair healthy.

Apply products. After you wash your beard, apply a moisturiser or an oil to keep it looking slick.

Style your beard. Finally, use a beard comb to complete your desired look. You can also use a small amount of wax to style your moustache.

BEARD PRODUCTS

BEARD OIL
Beard oil is essential for adding nutrients to your skin and hair. Beard hair is naturally brittle, so a little oil can help soften the hair and keep it in good shape.

BEARD MOISTURISER
No one likes a bristly beard. Keep your beard soft by applying a daily moisturiser to your face and neck.

BEARD BALM
Beard balm has a lot of the same benefits as beard oil, but it can also help to style your beard and make it look fuller. If you struggle to grow a thick-looking beard, then a beard balm could be your best friend!

BEARD WAX
Beard wax is perfect for taming stray hairs or styling a sassy moustache. It can help to keep your beard in shape if you are looking for a slick style. Don't go overboard on the wax though - a little goes a long way.

PART 4

GROWTH PROBLEMS AND SOLUTIONS

PATCHY GROWTH

Age matters - most men don't reach their peak beard growing abilities until they are over 25. If you're still younger, you might have to hold out a bit to grow a full beard.

Give it time - don't give up on growing your beard after just a few weeks. If it's looking patchy, it could just be that you need to be patient. It usually takes at least 3 months for a beard to reach its potential!

Exercise - Boost that all important testosterone by pumping some iron! Weight lifting is a great way to speed up your beard growth whilst also improving your overall fitness.

Diet - Vitamins and minerals are important for healthy beard growth. Eating foods rich in zinc, iron, vitamins B, C and D can help fix patchy beard growth!

SLOW GROWTH

Keep your face clean - A good skin care routine is vital for growing a beard. Wash your face regularly to prevent breakouts that might slow down growth.

Exfoliate -hair follicles will come through more easily on exfoliated skin. To speed up beard growth, try using a gentle scrub to remove dry skin twice a week.

Stressed? Try not to worry about your beard growth. Relax, take a deep breath, or meditate and you might see improved results!

FRIZZY GROWTH

Trim often - regular trimming is important for keeping rogue hairs at bay. Comb and trim your beard twice a week and cut back any unruly, long or frizzy hairs.
Keep it clean - washing your beard every day will keep it in good condition and prevent it from getting

too frizzy.

Use of products - beard oil and moisturising are essential for frizzy beards. Apply regularly to tackle the frizz!

Printed in Great Britain
by Amazon

32149989R00029

IT'S GROW TIME

Are you frustrated with your fuzzy beard growth? Want to get that manly look but don't know where to start?

This book is your complete guide to growing and grooming the beard you've always wanted.

Once you're feeling confident with your new bearded look, you can groom yourself into one of the many beard styles we've included in the book!

ISBN 9798414446156

90000

9 798414 446156